#CurlyGirl: A Coloring Book for Curly Girls

This edition published by SmoakHouse Publishing in 2019
www.lizzsmoak.com

Illustrations: Scarlett Fawn
Typeface Designs: Lizz Smoak
Cover Colorist: Jenny Morgan
Author Photo: Tara Beth Photography

For more products like this one visit: www.curlpowered.com

Designed in the United States of America

First Edition

#Curly Girl

Curly hair is hard work!

Whoever thought up curly hair took the meaning of "Beauty is Pain" to a whole new level!

Curly girls spend so much time (and money) on their hair that I thought it would be a nice change to focus on the fun curly girls get to have with their gorgeous, often too-touchable springy locks.

My collection of original illustrations and witty quotes were designed with you in mind. Let yourself escape and relax into the art of coloring and build in this modern form of art and meditation into your weekly wash day habits.

Name your girls, make them funky or share them with a curly friend. Whatever you desire, grab your pens, pencils, markers or crayons and enjoy the therapeutic effects of coloring your newfound circle of curly girls.

I'm happy you found this tool and welcome you into my world of curly fun. I'm wishing you many days of inspired coloring.

 CURLPILLOWS

 MAJORMESS123

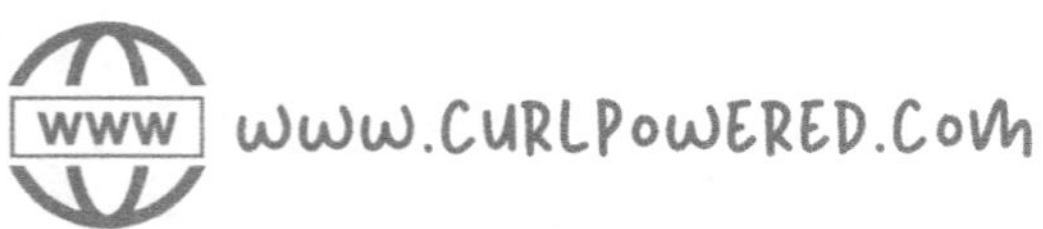 WWW.CURLPOWERED.COM

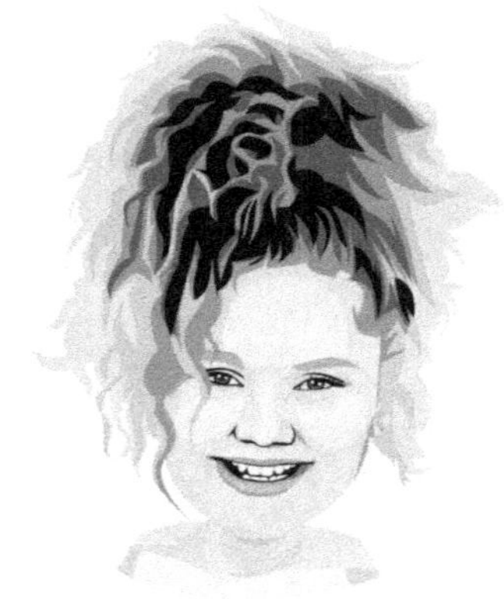

xoxo,

Sophia Allen

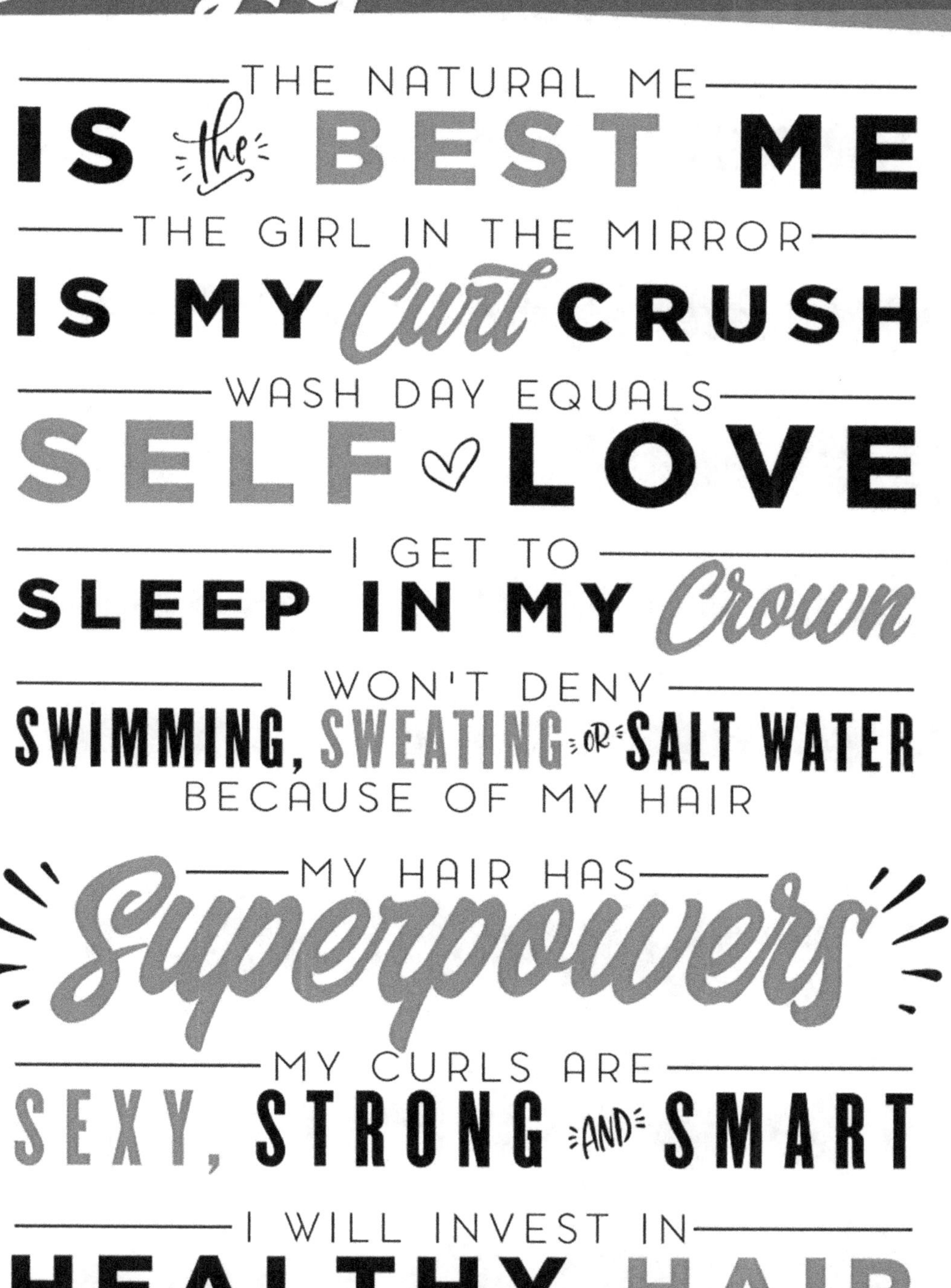

Curly Girl MANIFESTO
THE NATURAL ME
IS the BEST ME
THE GIRL IN THE MIRROR
IS MY Curl CRUSH
WASH DAY EQUALS
SELF LOVE
I GET TO
SLEEP IN MY Crown
I WON'T DENY
SWIMMING, SWEATING or SALT WATER
BECAUSE OF MY HAIR
MY HAIR HAS
Superpowers
MY CURLS ARE
SEXY, STRONG AND SMART
I WILL INVEST IN
HEALTHY HAIR
I WILL SHOW MY CURLS
GRATITUDE
I AM Curl POWERED

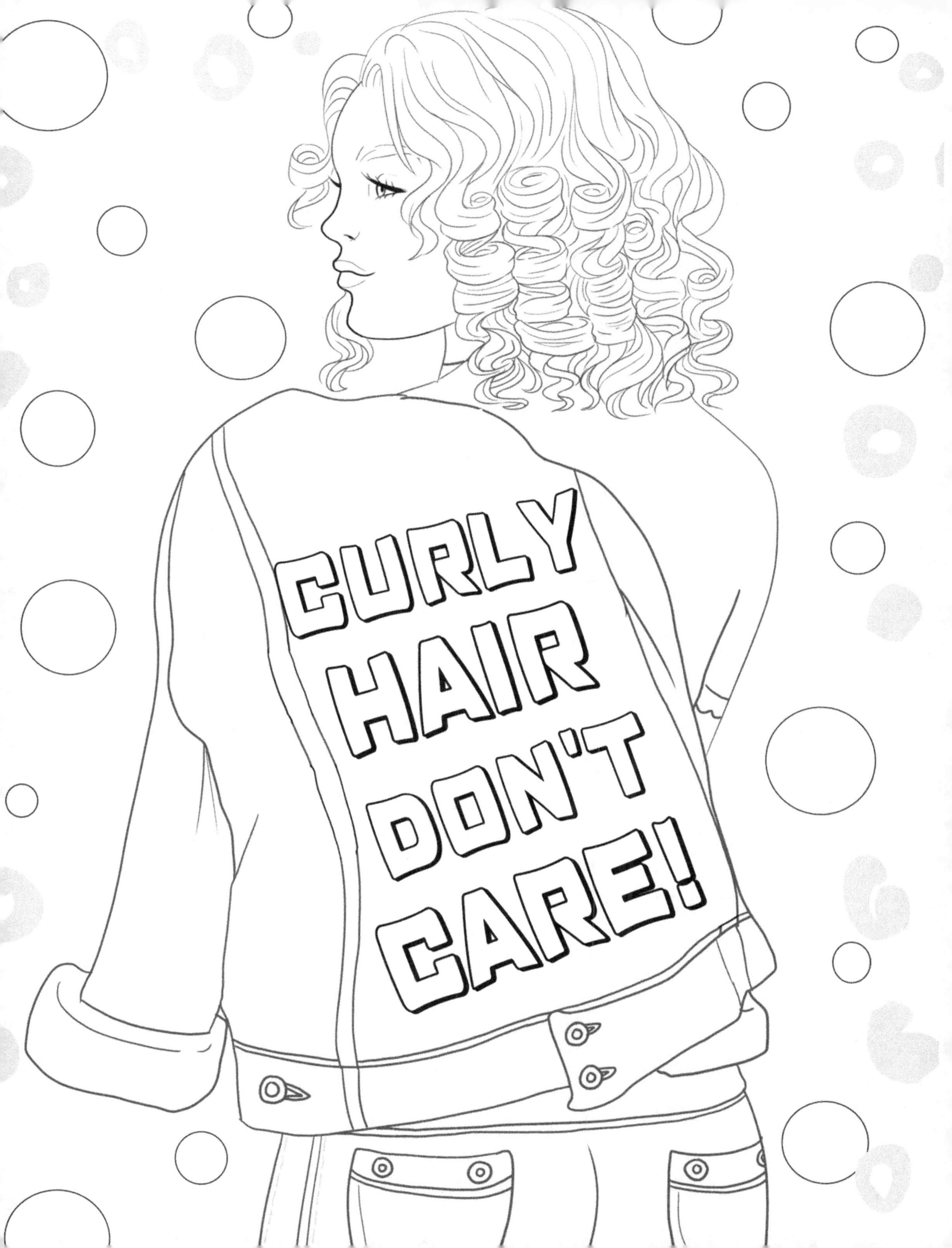

CURLY
HAIR
DON'T
CARE!

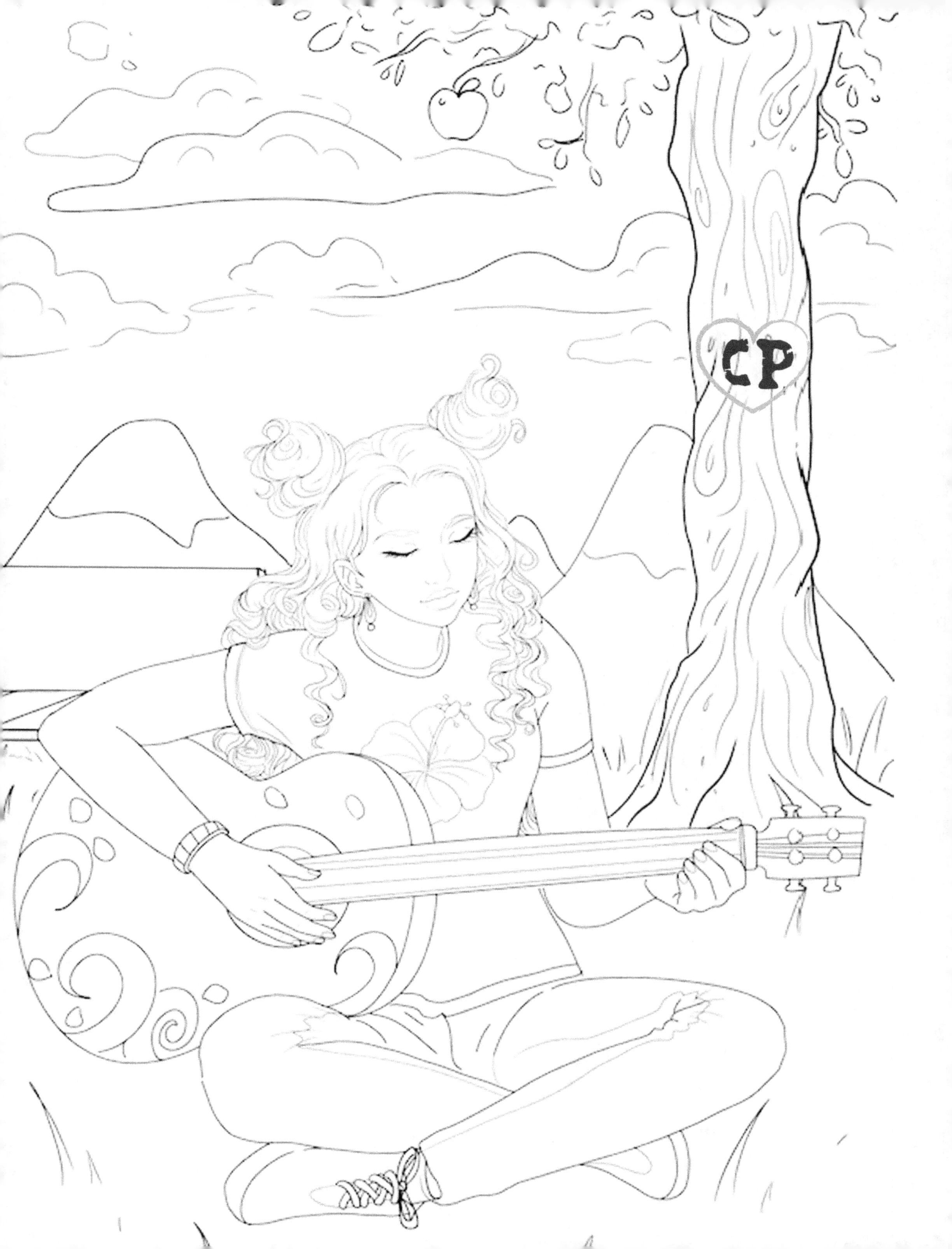
CP

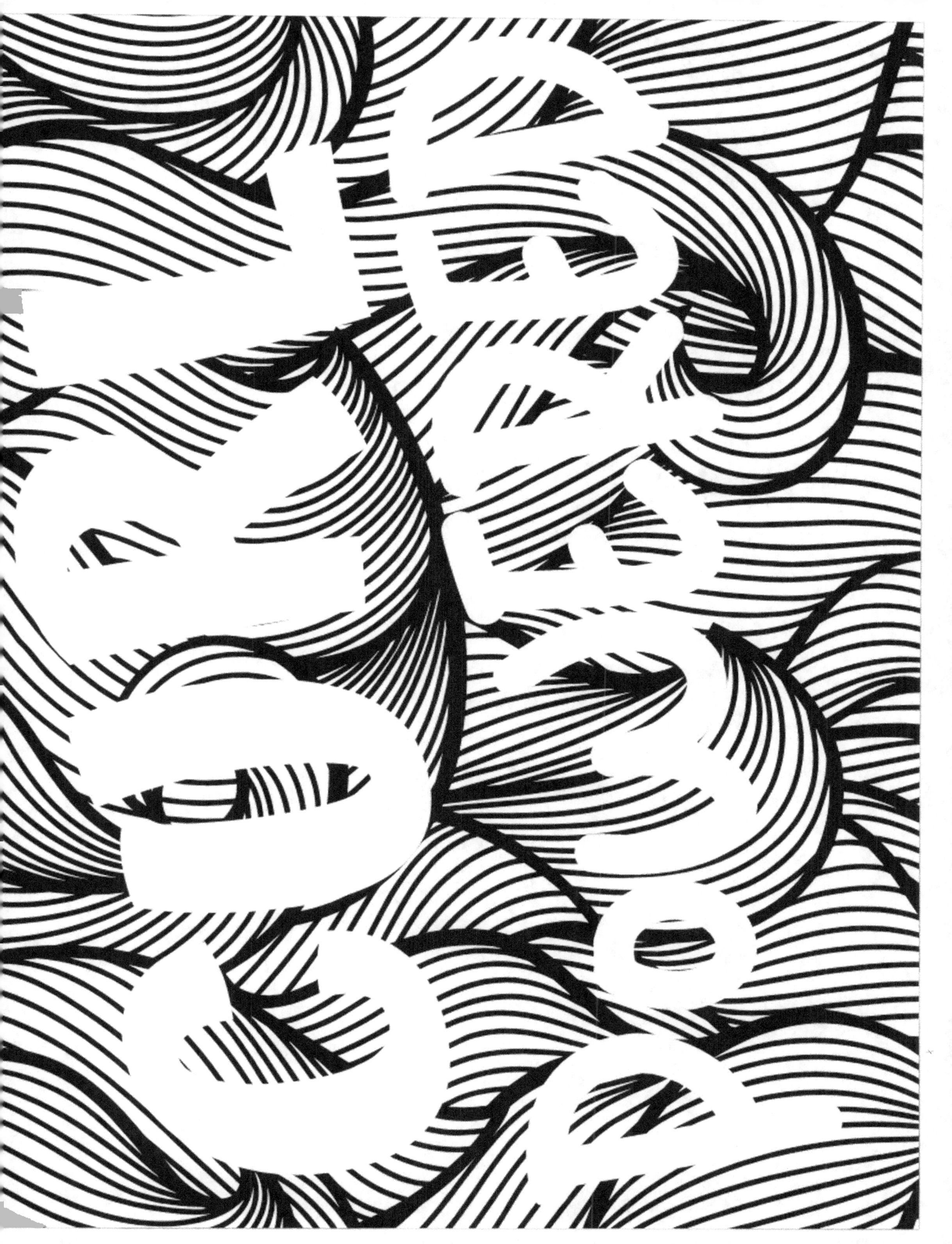

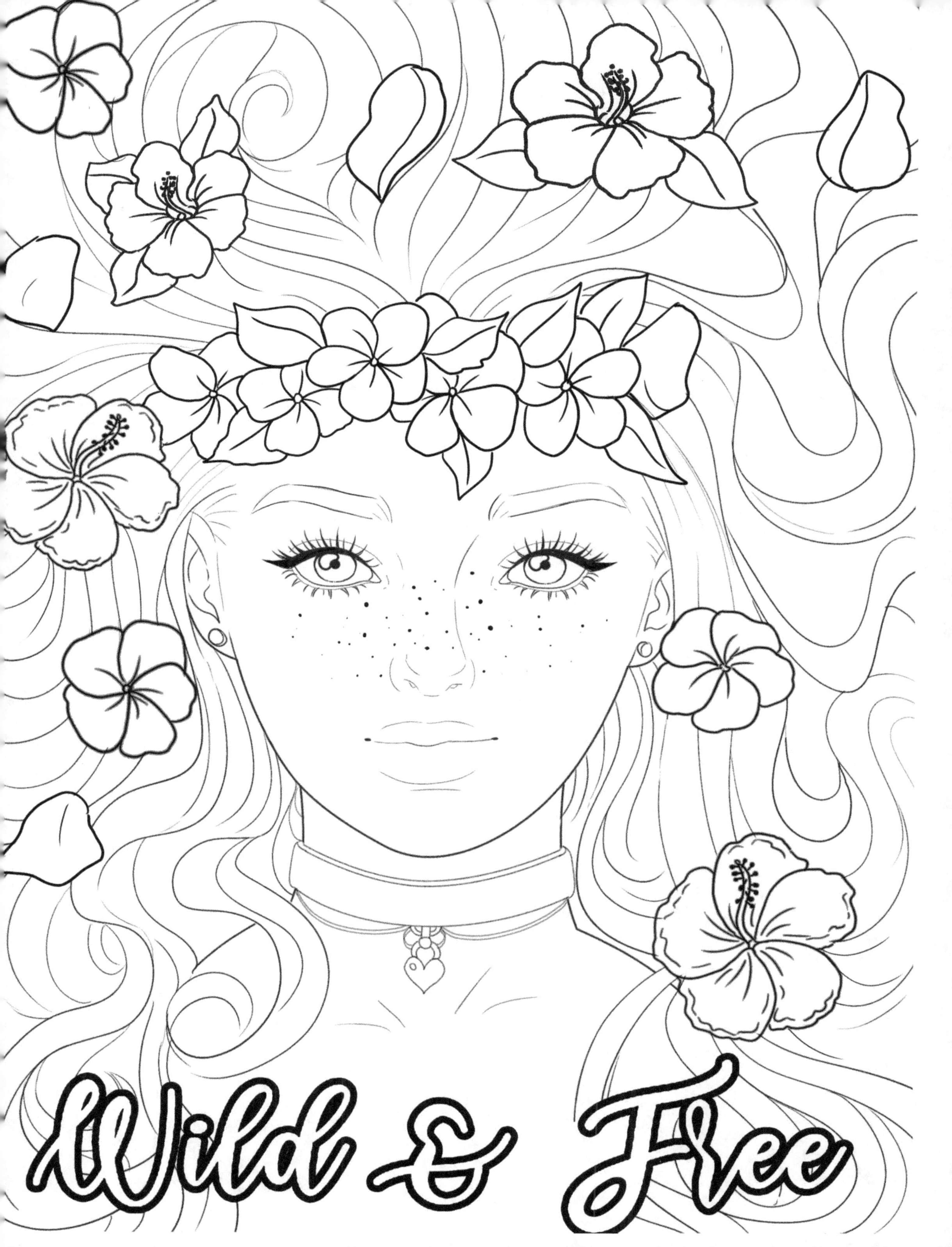
Wild & Free

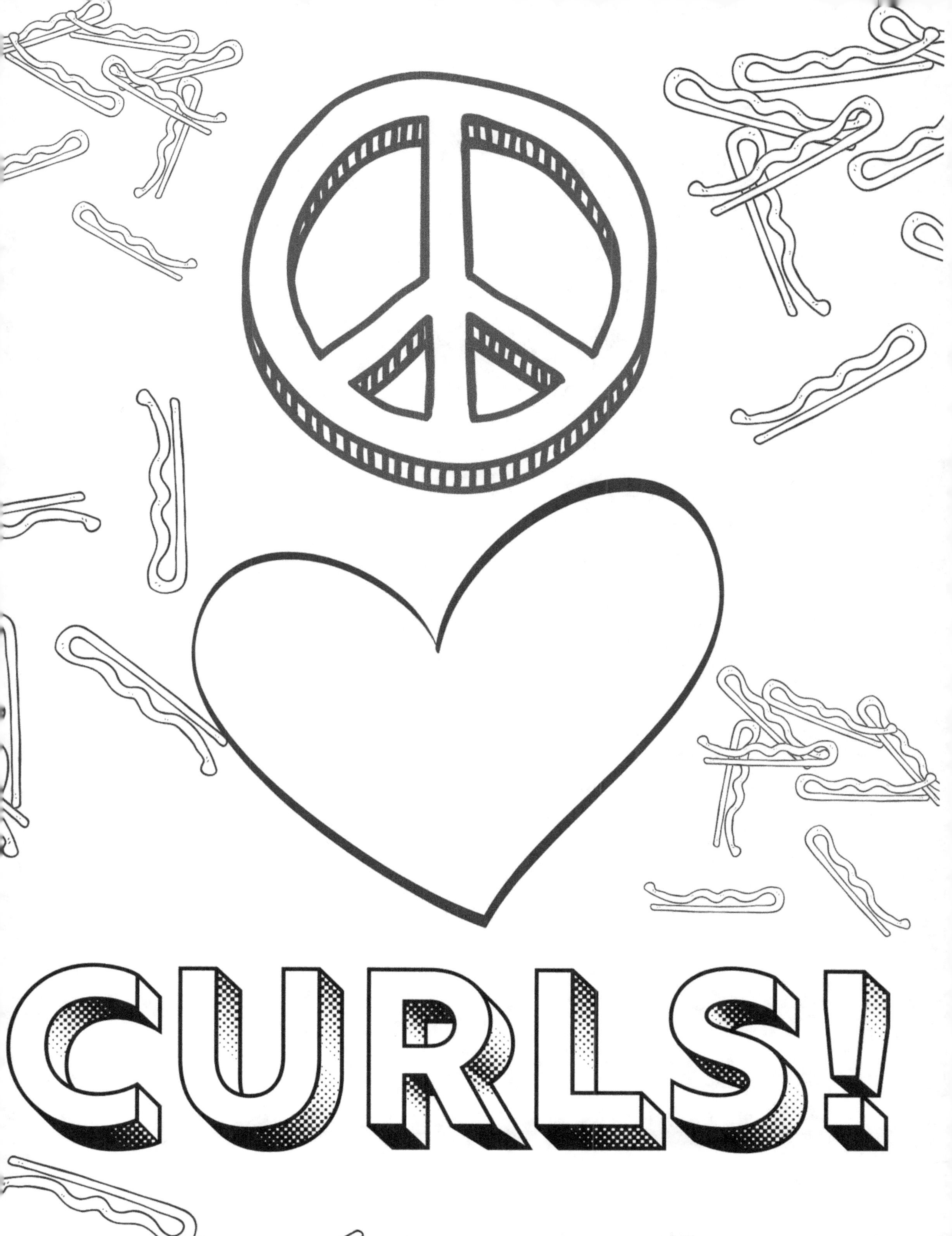

CURLS!

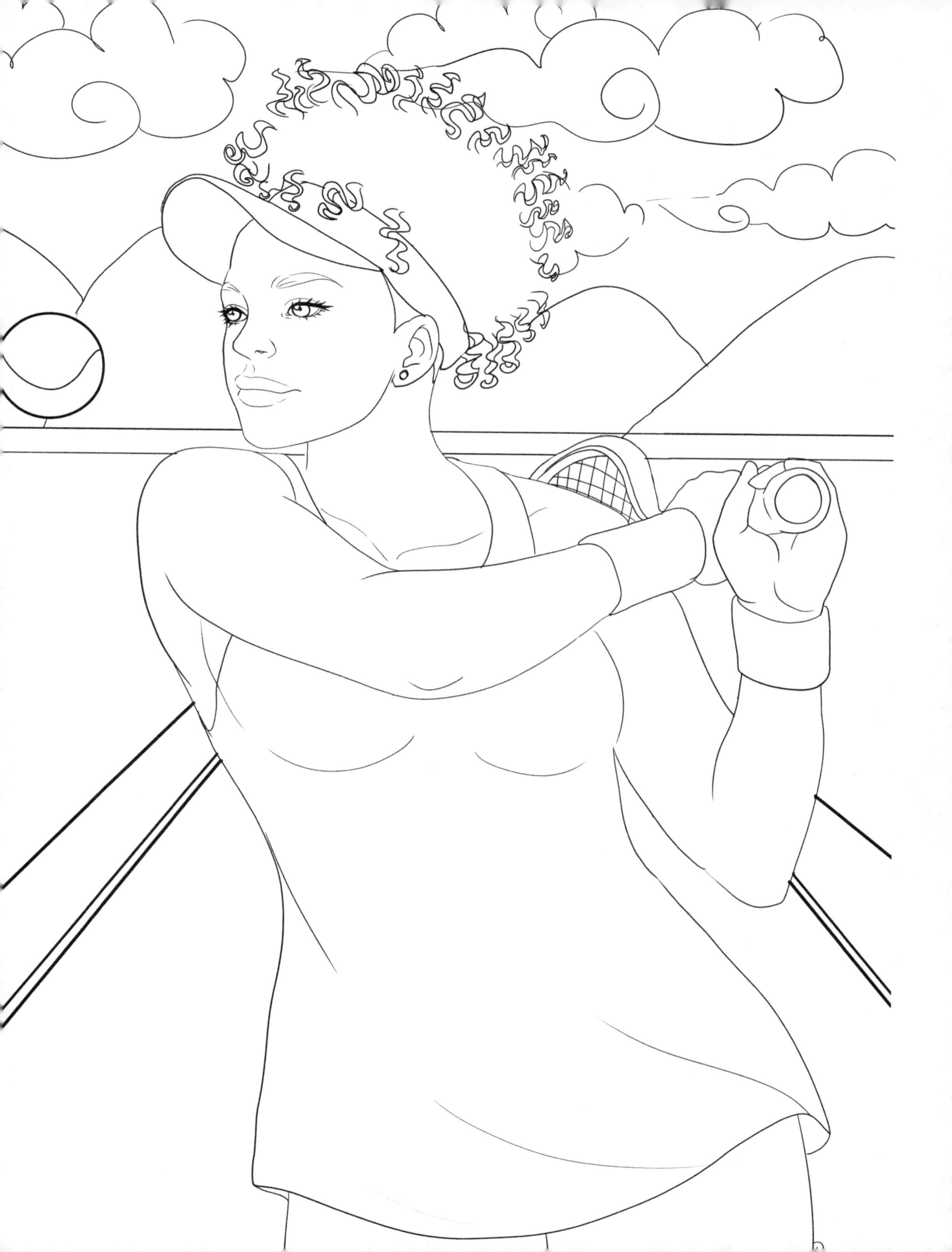

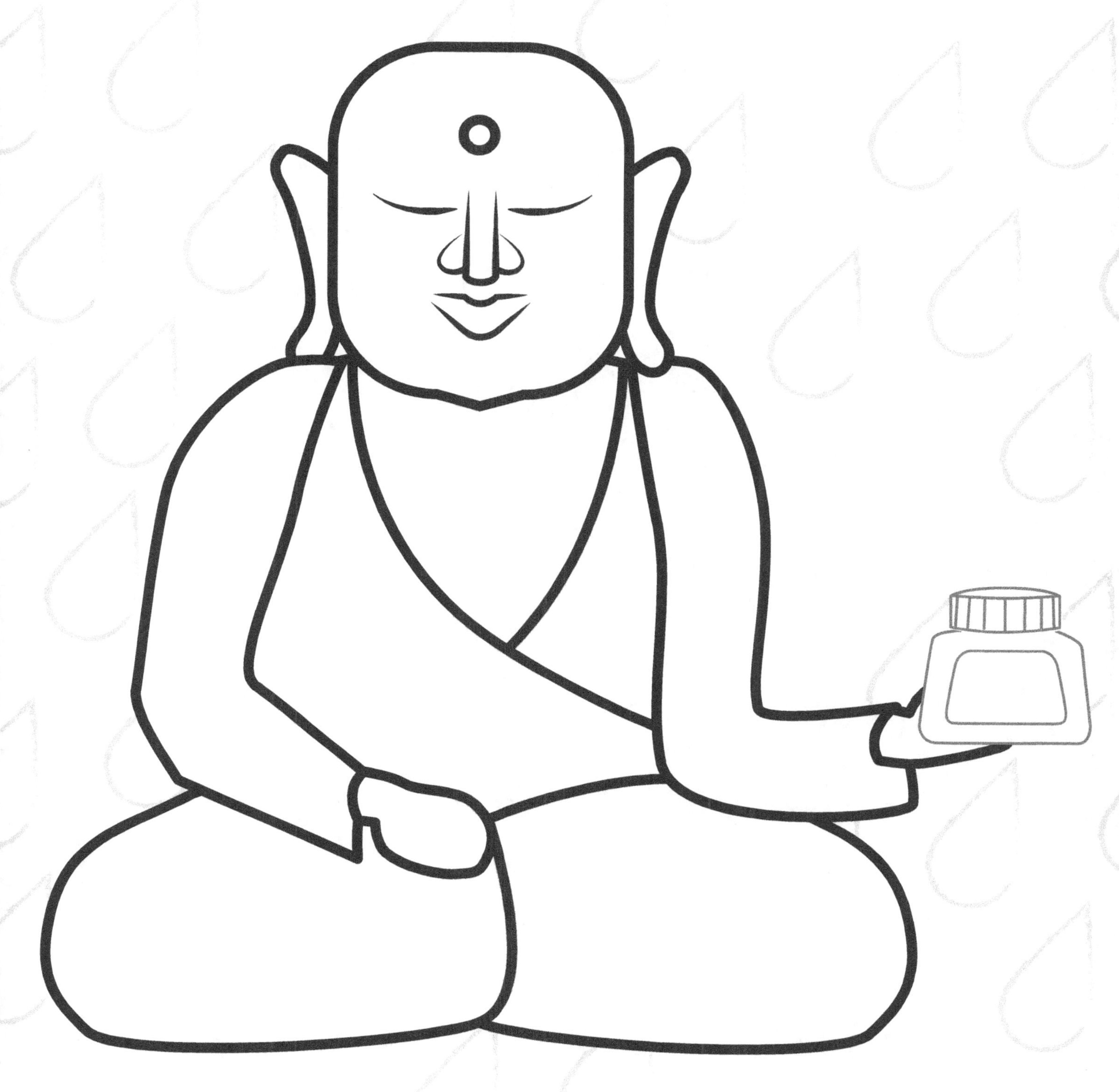

1. Wash Hair
2. Hope for the Best

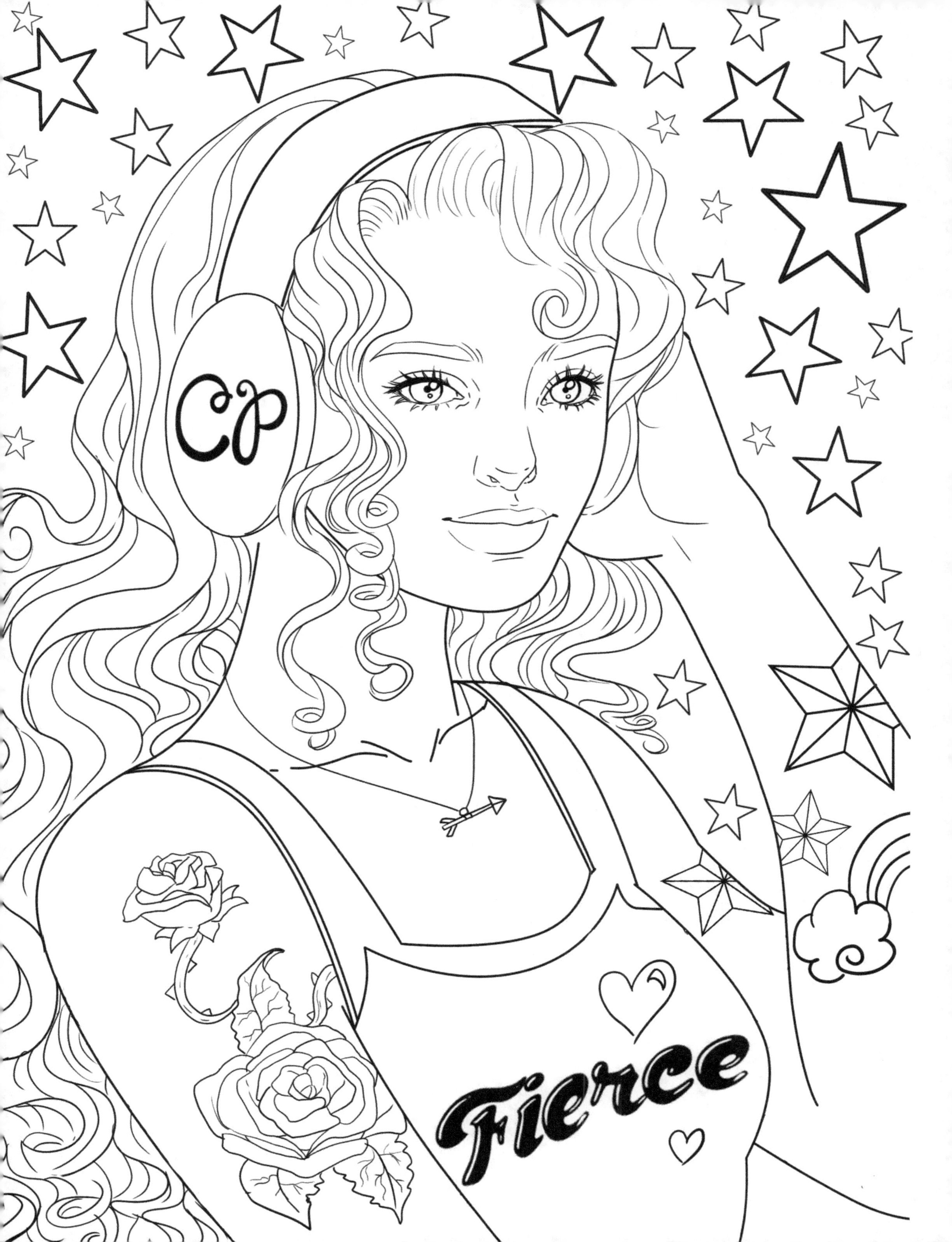
CP
Fierce

Big Hair

Big Dreams ♡

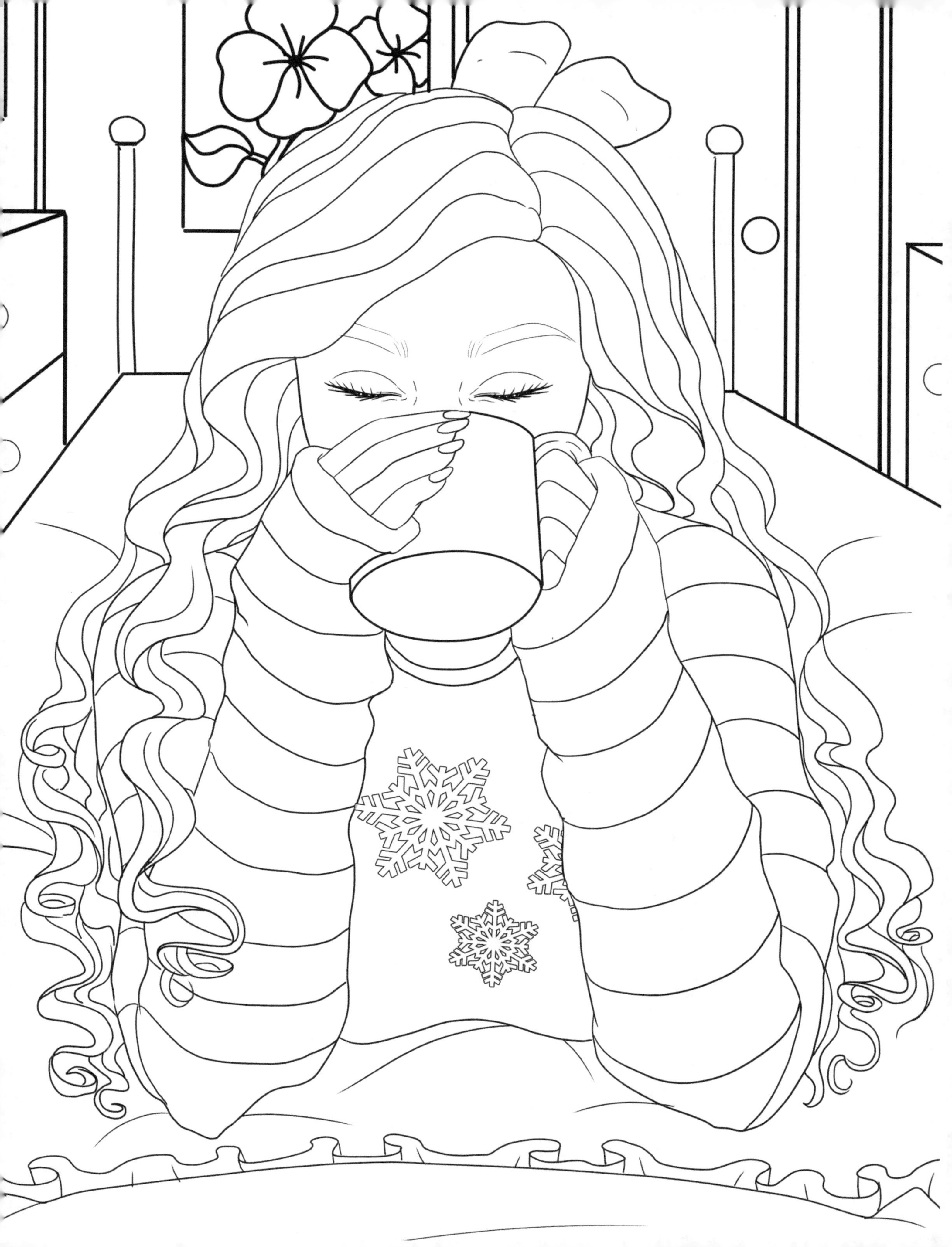

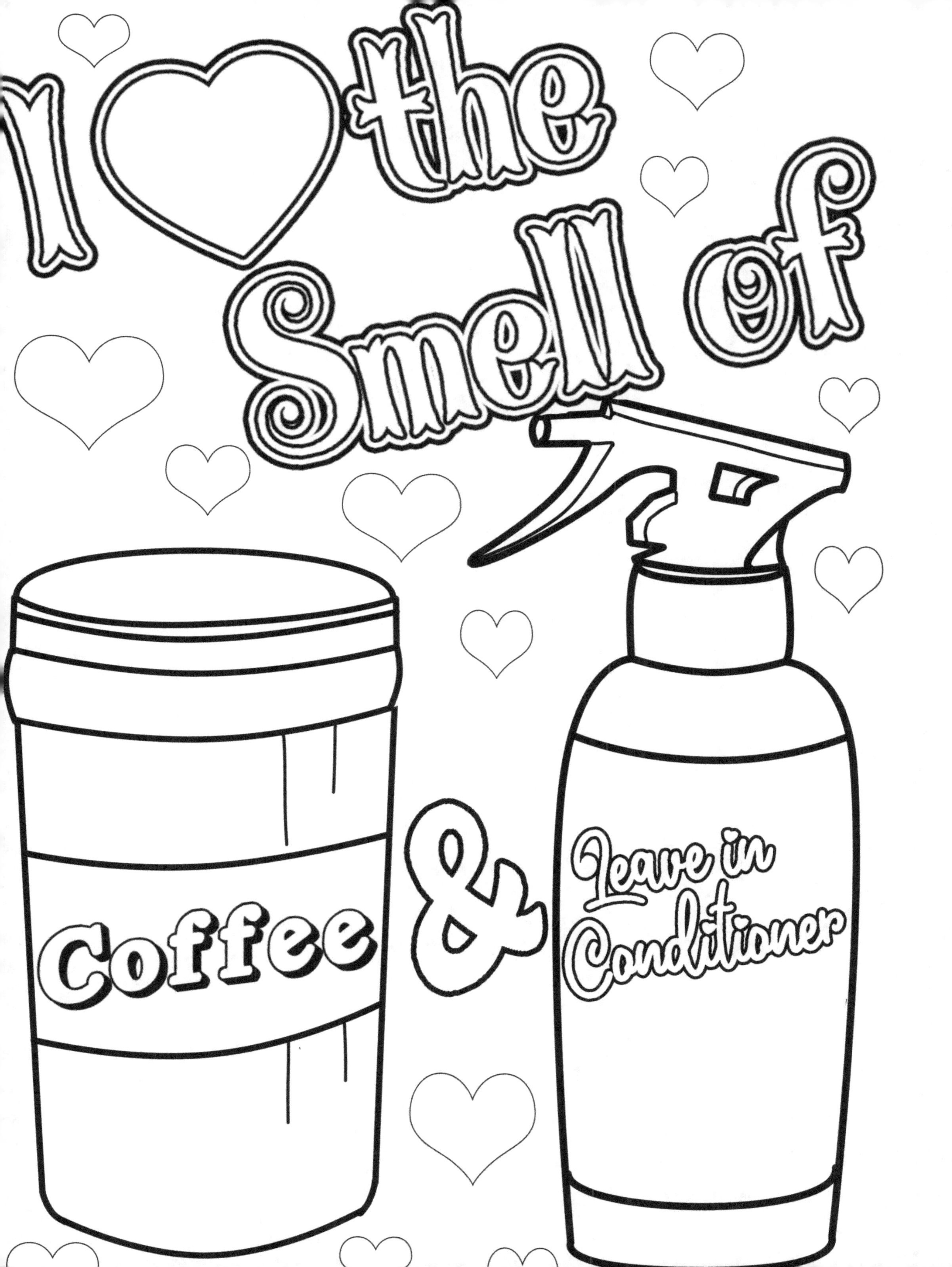

I ♥ the smell of
Coffee & Leave in Conditioner

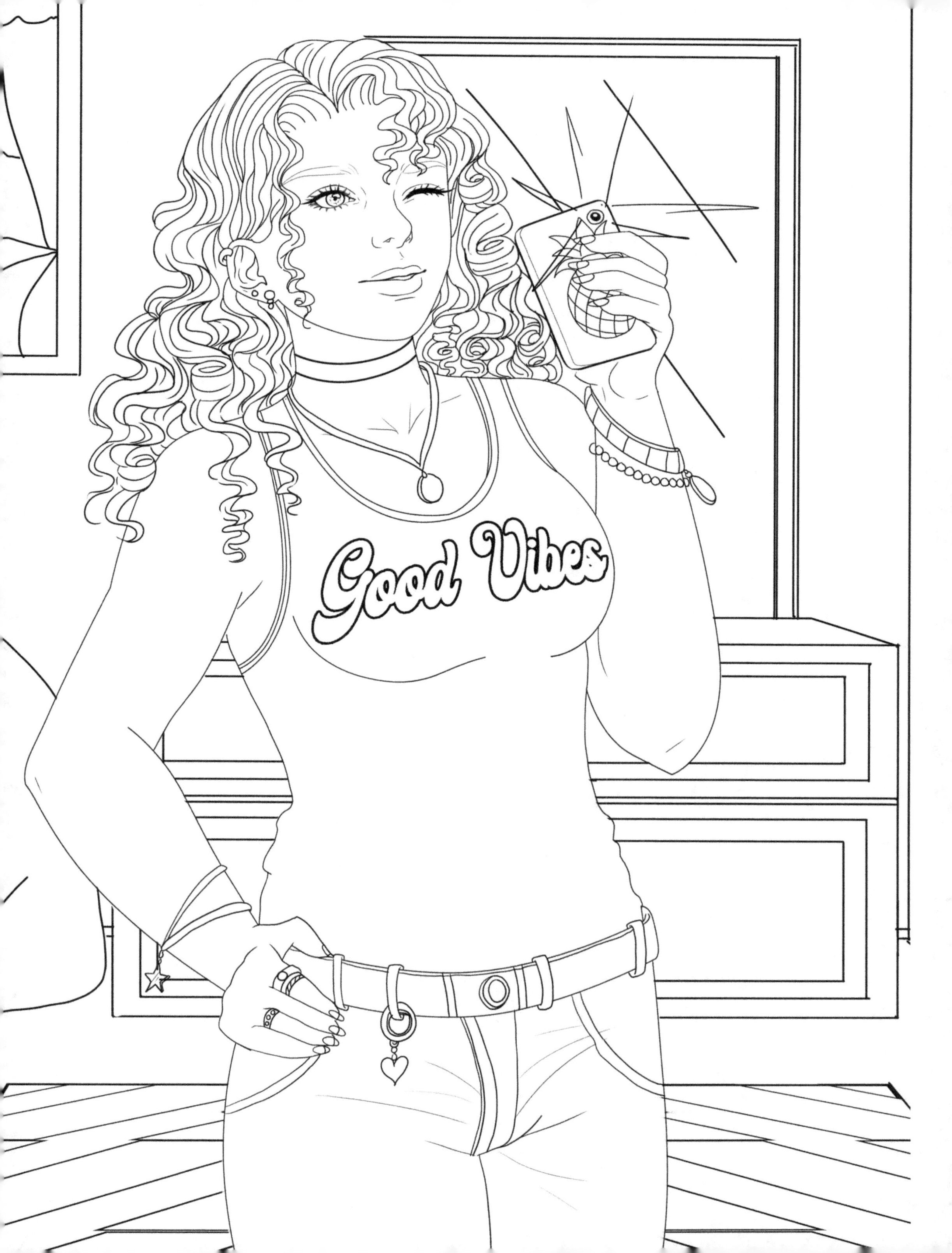
Good Vibes

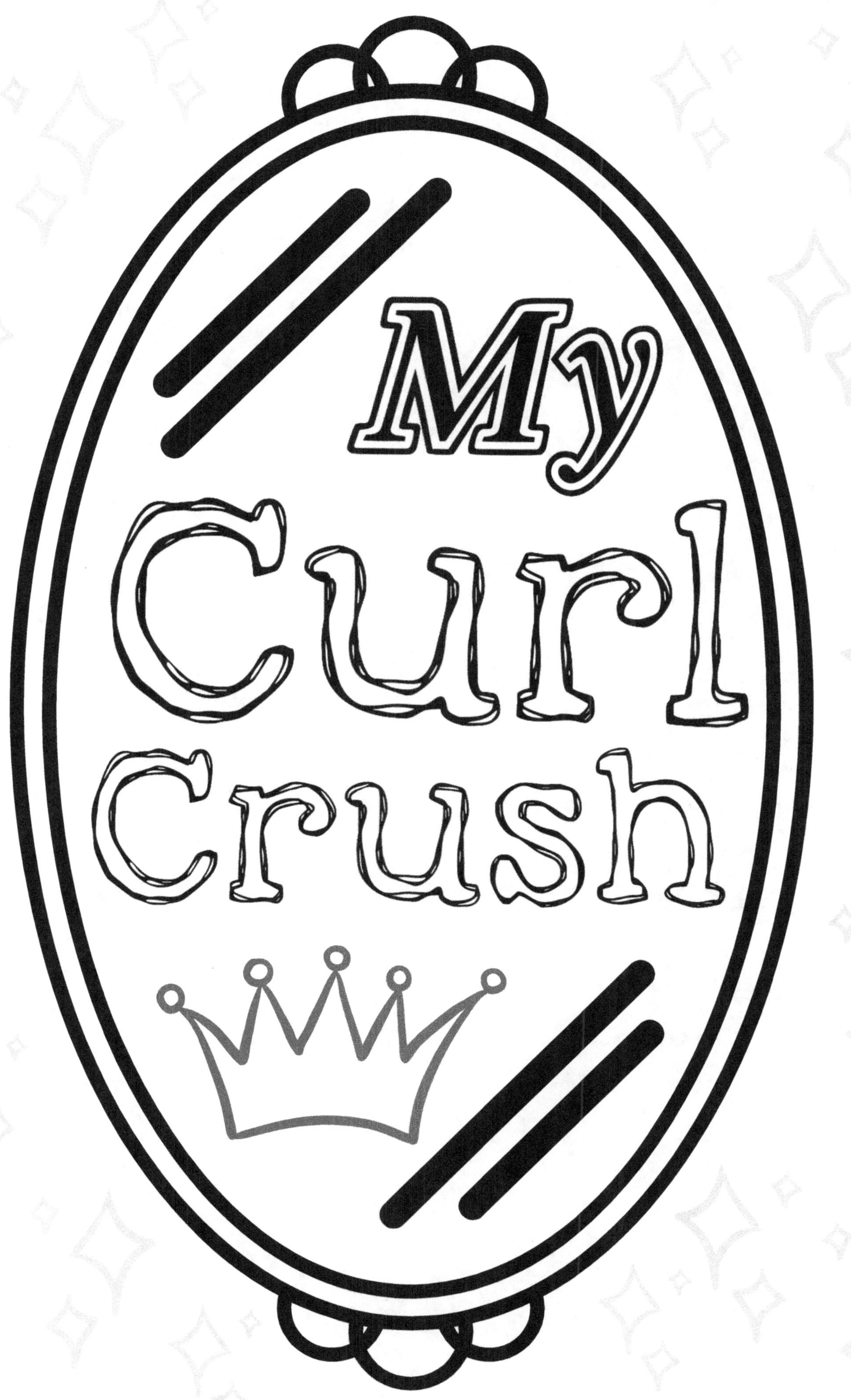
My
Curl
Crush

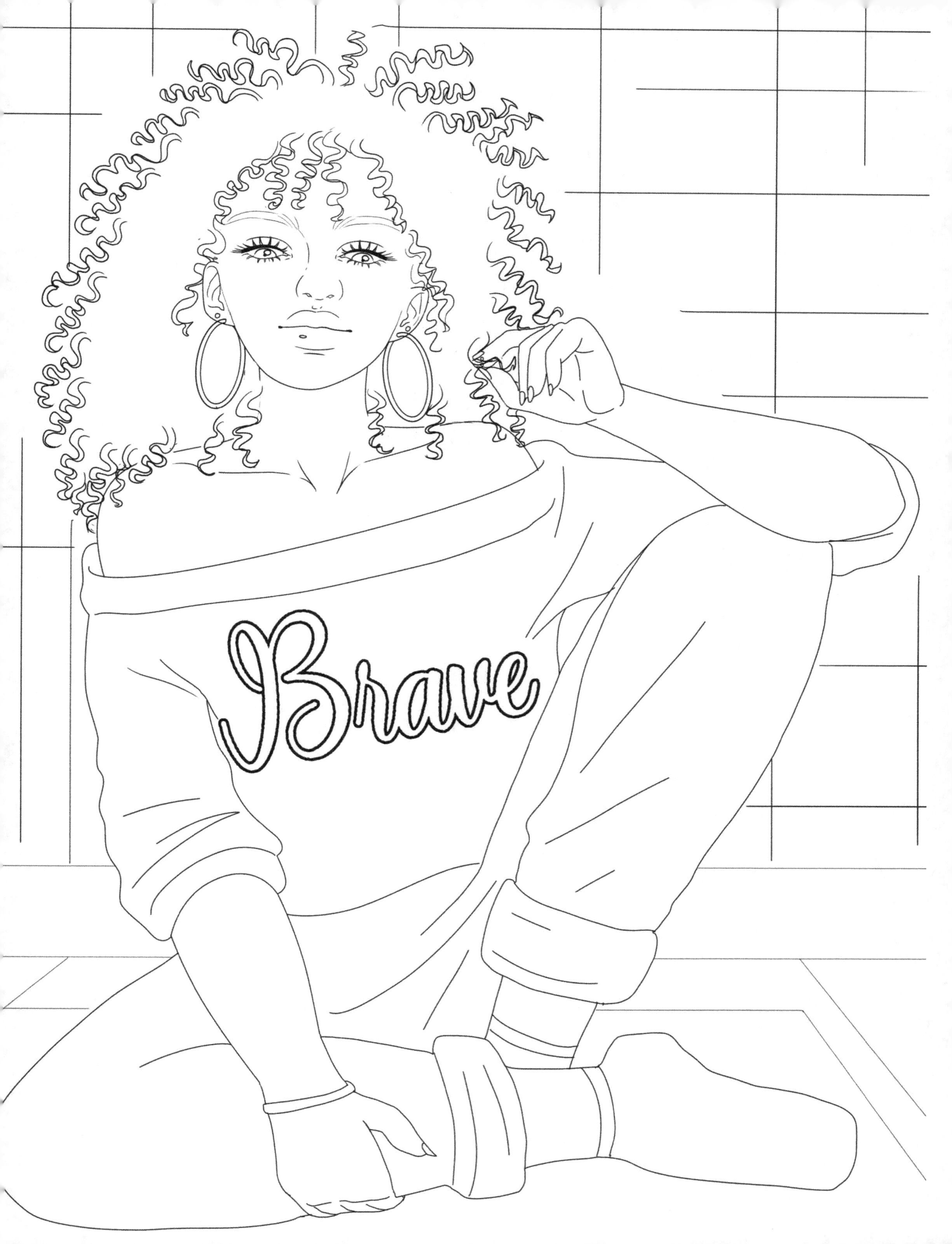
Brave

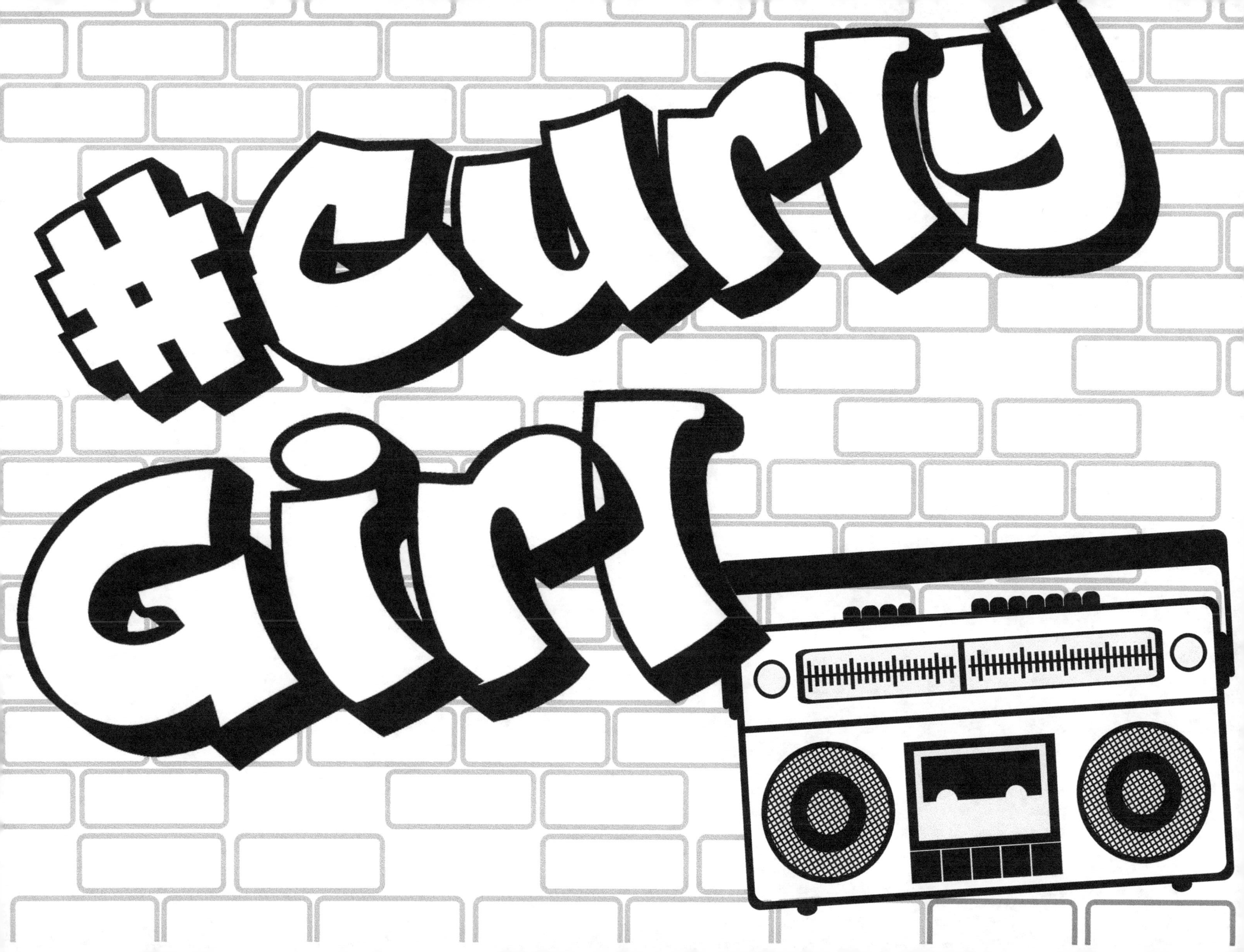
#curly
Girl

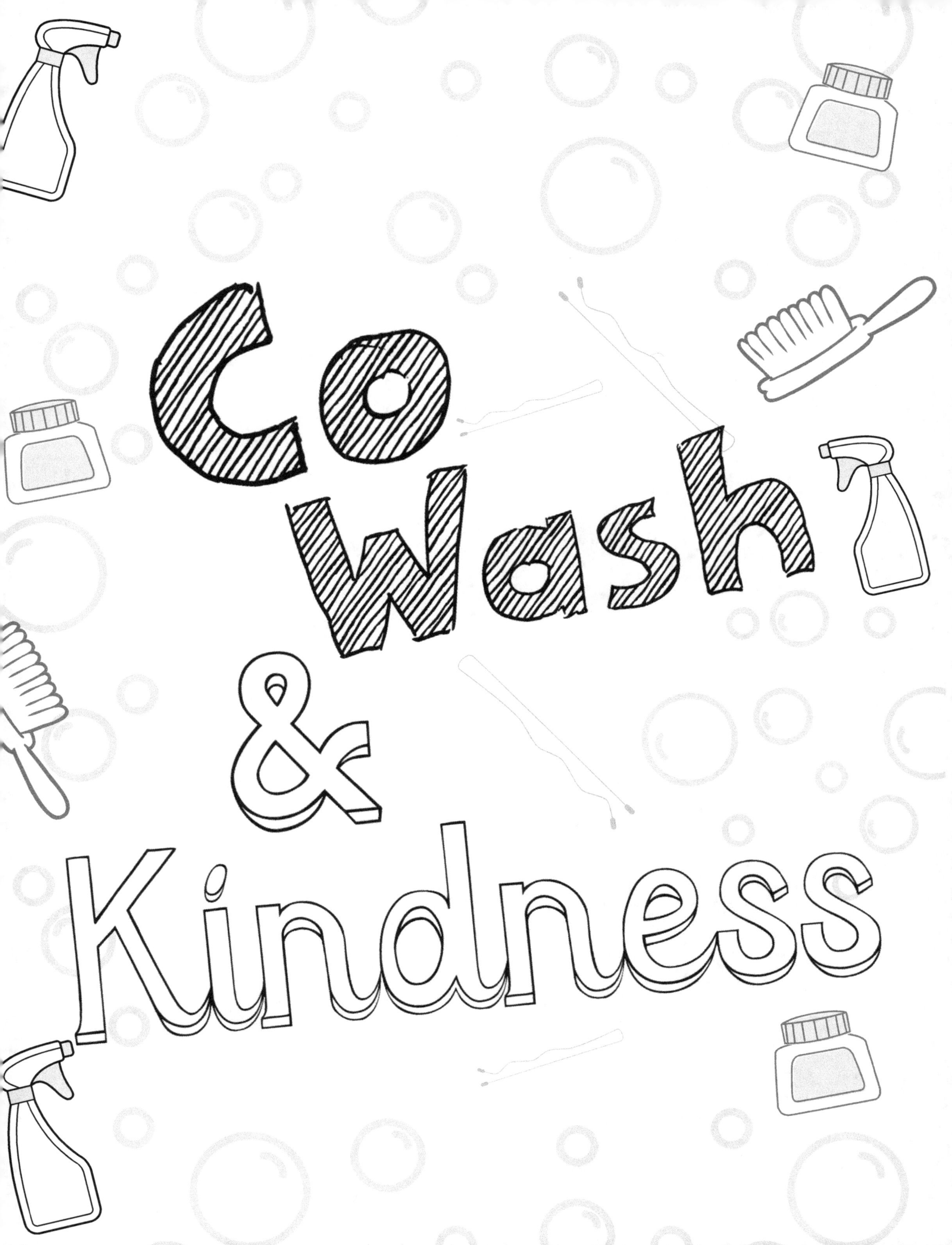

Co
Wash
&
Kindness

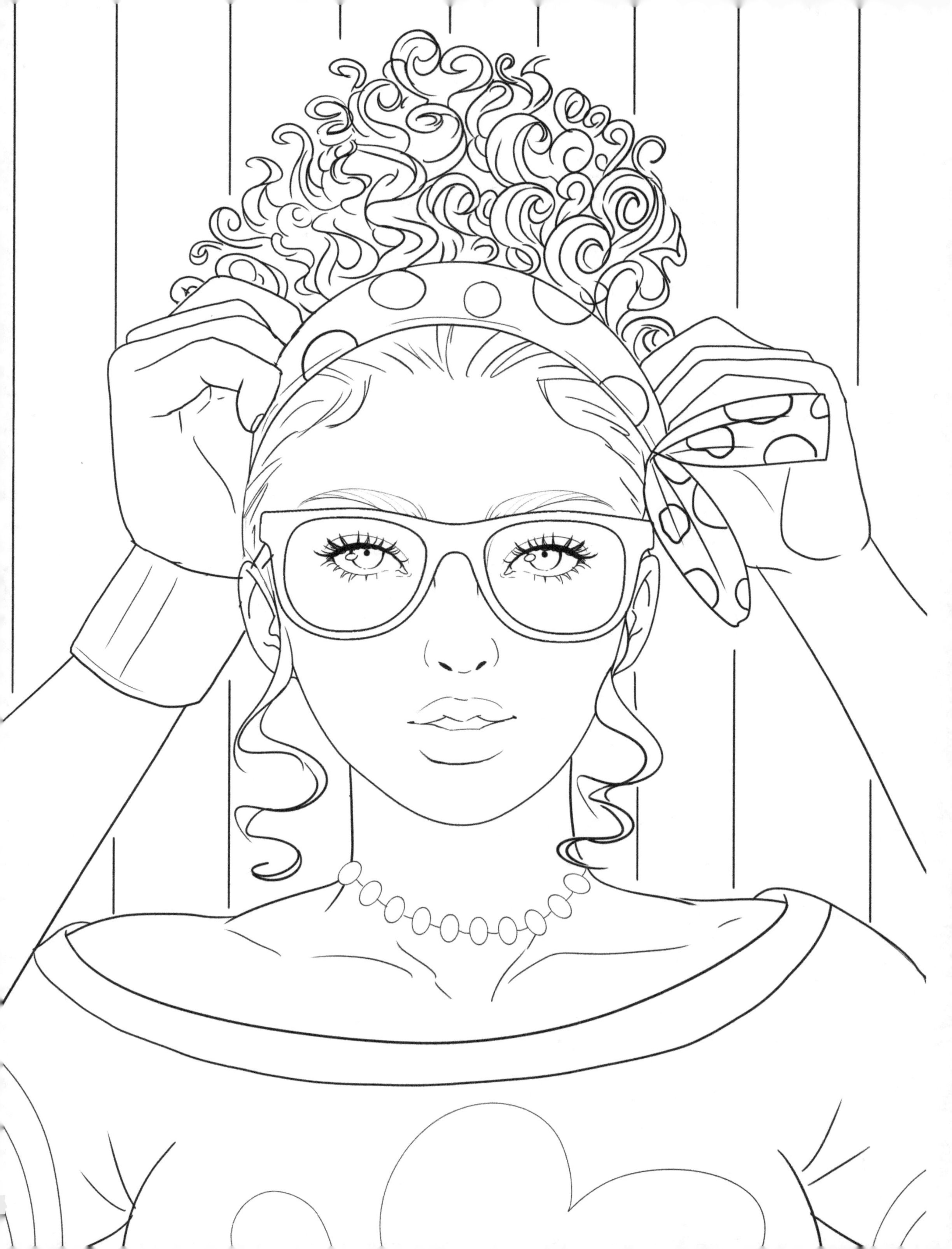

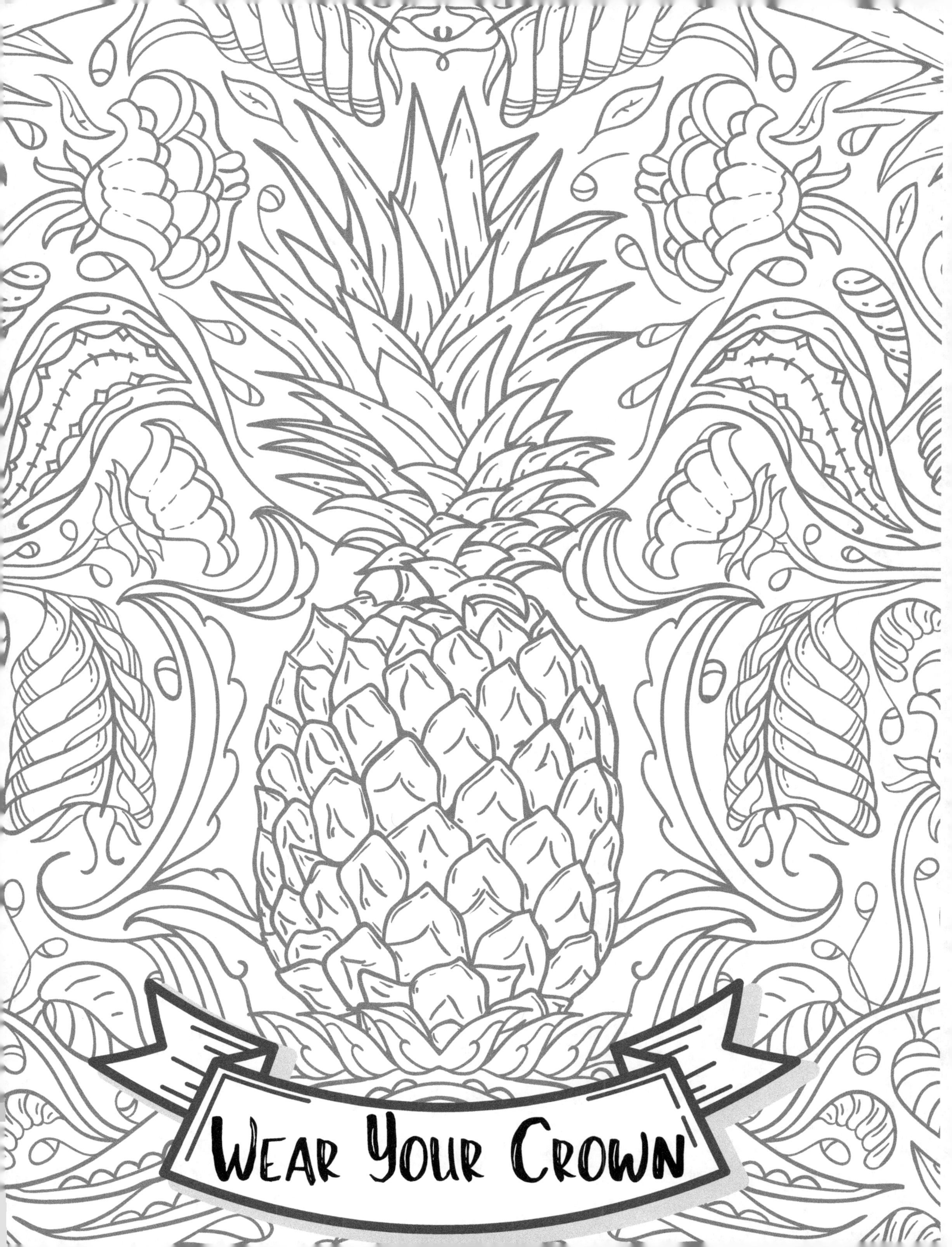

Wear Your Crown

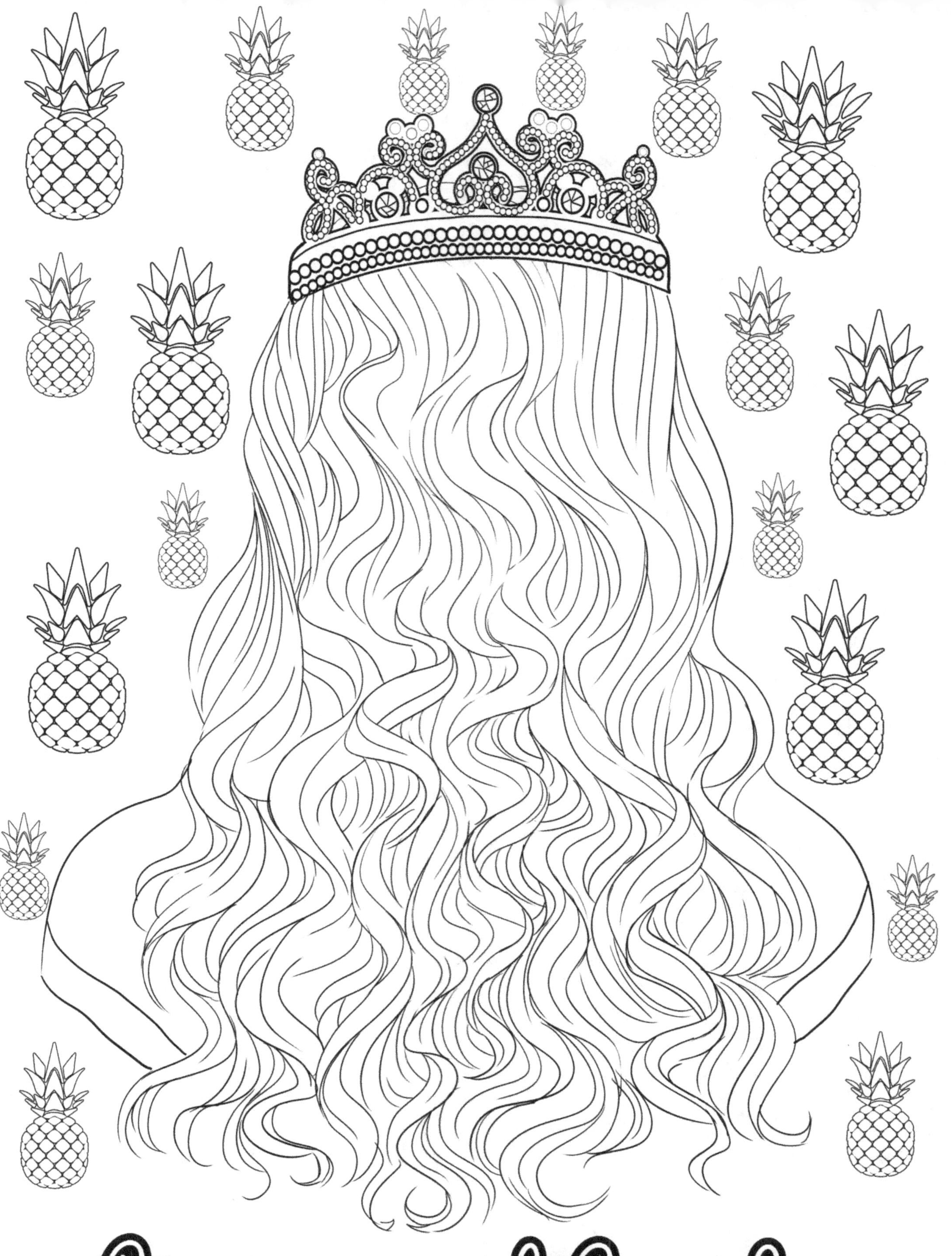

Crown of Curls

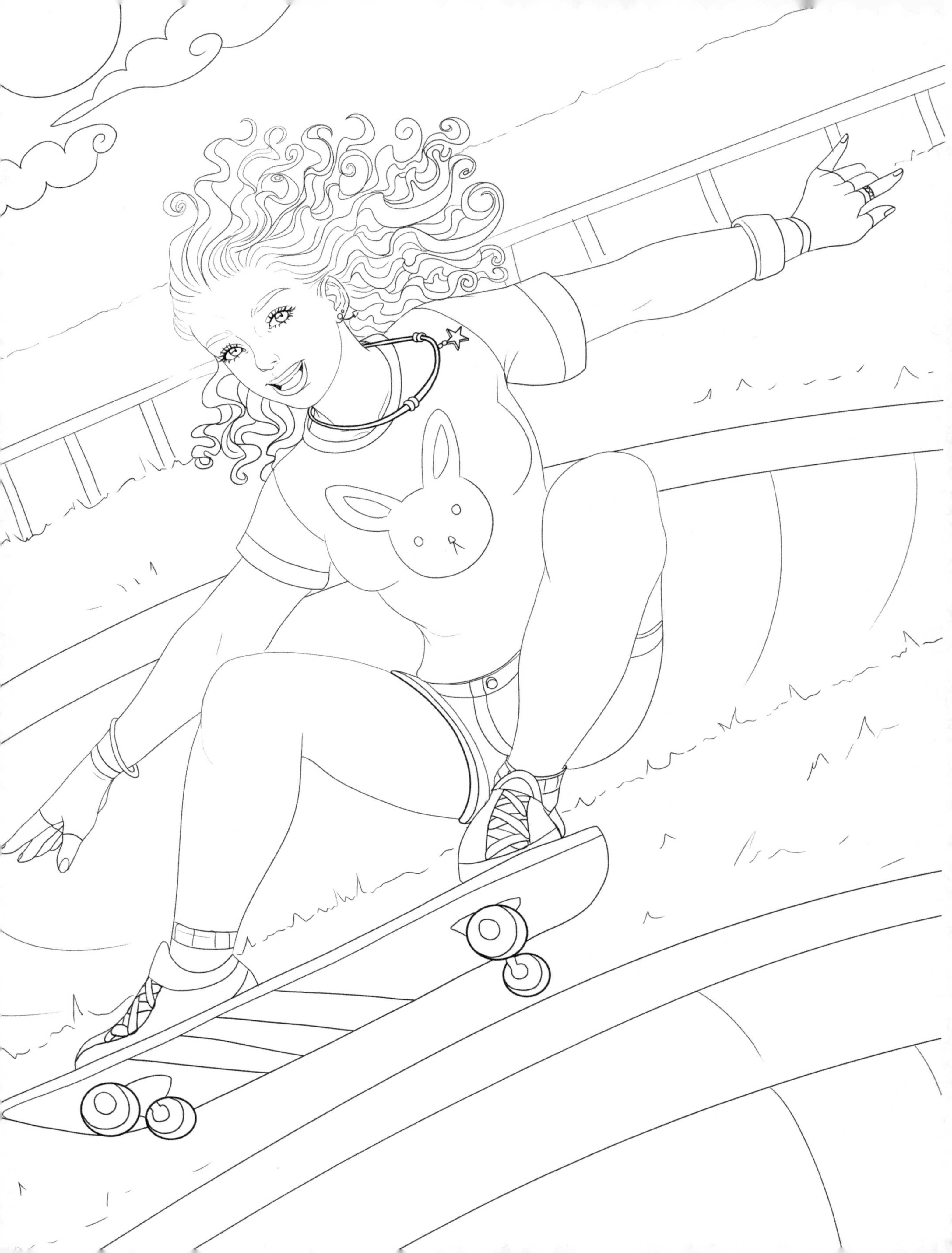

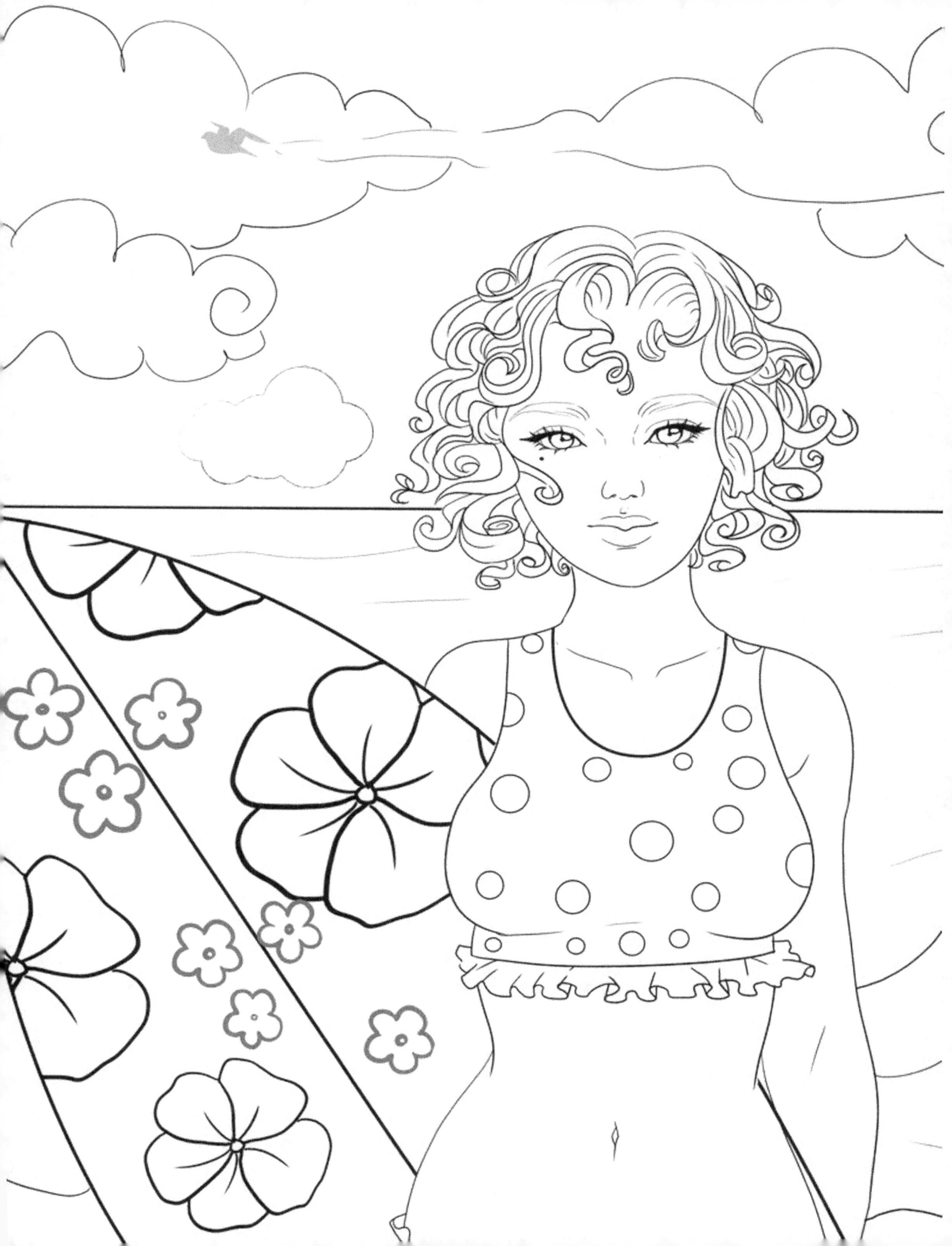

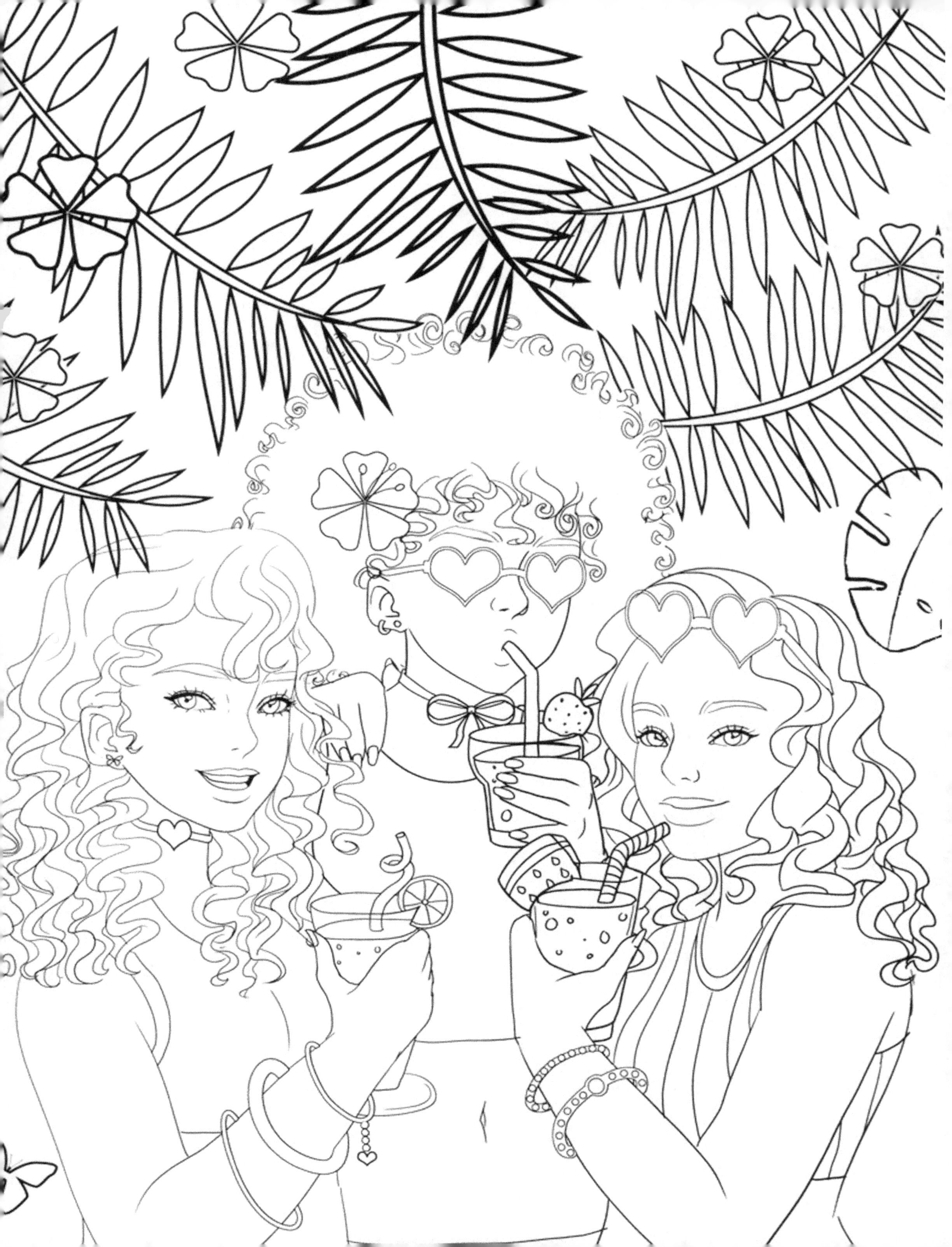